Copyright © 2023 di

All rights reserved

This book is licensed for personal use only.

The book cannot be sold or transferred to third parties.

Wall Pilates Workouts for Women

DISCLAIMER

This is a general physical education book, all information included is intended for healthy adults 18 and older. The intention of this book is purely informational and educational in nature and is not intended to provide medical advice. Consult your doctor before starting any sporting activity and any type of food plan. There may be risks associated with participating in the activities mentioned in this book for people in poor physical and/or mental health.

For this reason we discourage the use of the information contained in this book and participation in the activities described if you are in a precarious physical condition or come from a pre-existing condition of physical or mental discomfort. If you decide to participate in these activities, you choose to do so knowingly and voluntarily on your own free initiative aware of all the risks associated with these activities.

Introduction

The Rise of Wall Pilates

In a world where fitness trends come and go, there's something uniquely enduring about Pilates. From its humble beginnings in the early 20th century with Joseph Pilates, this form of exercise has grown and adapted, finding its way into the routines of elite athletes, celebrities, and women everywhere looking to enhance their strength, flexibility, and mind-body connection.

But, as with any discipline that stands the test of time, innovation is key. Enter Wall Pilates.

Wall Pilates emerged as an answer to modern needs. In the bustling pace of the 21st century, not everyone has the luxury of expansive spaces or specialized equipment. Our homes became our gyms, our sanctuaries. And in this transformation, the wall, something so fundamental and often overlooked, became a potent tool for transformation.

What makes Wall Pilates so alluring, especially to women, is its marriage of accessibility and potency. You don't need an elaborate setup or even a lot of room. A wall and a dedication to self-betterment are all that's required.

Many women found themselves gravitating towards Wall Pilates as it not only catered to their physical needs—like toning, improving posture, and enhancing core strength—but also their emotional and mental needs. In a society that often feels like it's pulling us in a million directions, there's solace in the simplicity and focus Wall Pilates demands.

The beauty of Wall Pilates, beyond its effectiveness, is its inclusivity. Whether you're a seasoned fitness enthusiast, a busy mom seeking some 'me time', or someone just starting their journey towards a healthier self, Wall Pilates meets you where you are. It's more than just a trend; it's a movement. A movement rooted in the principles of traditional Pilates but modernized for the woman of today. A movement that champions self-love, empowerment, and growth, all with the support of a simple wall.

So, as we delve deeper into this book, we'll explore the intricate techniques, the transformative exercises, and the powerful stories of women who've changed their lives one Wall Pilates session at a time. Welcome to the world of Wall Pilates, a world where every woman can rise, thrive, and shine.

Embracing the Struggles and Transforming Lives

Life's challenges are multifaceted, and for many women, they manifest in both physical and emotional realms. The stories of struggles are as varied as they are many: from postpartum bodies yearning to find their former strength, to professionals battling the slouch of hours spent at a desk, to women of all ages fighting against the tug of gravity and time. Amidst these battles, Wall Pilates has emerged as a beacon of hope and transformation.

At first glance, it might seem curious that a workout regimen involving a wall could tackle these deeply personal and complex struggles. But, as with many profound journeys, the magic of Wall Pilates is hidden within its simplicity.

The Physical Struggles:

For those suffering from posture-related issues, the wall serves as an immediate feedback tool. Unlike other workouts where it's easy to cheat or adjust unconsciously, the wall is unyielding and honest. It tells you when you're leaning too much, when you're not aligned, and when you're perfectly poised.

Then there are the weight-related challenges. The resistance and support of the wall allow for an intensity of workout that burns calories and tones muscles without the need for weights or other equipment. Every push, pull, and stretch is amplified, making each session both challenging and rewarding.

The Emotional and Mental Struggles:

But Wall Pilates isn't just about the physical. It's a deeply emotional and mental practice. For women feeling overwhelmed, each session is an opportunity to reconnect with oneself. The wall, in many ways, mirrors life's challenges. It's unyielding and steadfast. But, with time, patience, and persistence, we learn to work with it, mold ourselves against it, and eventually use it to elevate ourselves.

There's a meditative quality to Wall Pilates. As you press against the wall, you're not just pushing against a physical barrier but also against self-doubt, against societal pressures, against internalized critiques. And as you peel away from the wall, stretch, and open up, it's symbolic of breaking free, of embracing one's potential, of soaring.

Transforming Lives:

Clara's Journey: At 32, post-childbirth, Clara felt like she was trapped in a body she didn't recognize. The challenges of motherhood, coupled with the physical changes she underwent, made her feel disconnected. Wall Pilates became her sanctuary. With every session, she felt a growing bond with her body, and within months, not only did she see physical changes, but she also found an empowering confidence that permeated every aspect of her life.

Lydia's Renewal: Lydia, a 45-year-old executive, was on the verge of resigning herself to a life of chronic back pain due to long hours at her desk job. She stumbled upon Wall Pilates almost by accident. The exercises seemed so simple, yet the results were profound. The wall helped her correct her posture, alleviating her pain. More than that, it reignited a passion and zest for life that she thought she had lost.

Their stories, while unique, echo a shared sentiment: Wall Pilates is more than a workout; it's a lifeline. It's a dance of strength and vulnerability, of challenge and triumph, of embracing struggles and, in doing so, transforming lives.

Why Wall Pilates is Perfect for Women

In a world saturated with workout regimens, fad diets, and ever-evolving fitness gadgets, Wall Pilates stands out, especially for women. But what makes this method so uniquely suited for the female form and psyche? Let's delve into the intricacies of Wall Pilates and why it resonates deeply with women around the globe.

1. Adaptable to Every Life Stage:

Whether navigating the changes that come with puberty, pregnancy, or menopause, a woman's body is in constant flux. Wall Pilates offers adaptable routines that can cater to these varied physical states, ensuring that a woman feels supported and challenged in every phase of her life.

2. Strength and Grace Combined:

Traditionally, workouts have been divided into two categories: those that offer strength and those that promise grace. Wall Pilates merges the two. The resistance of the wall allows for muscle building and toning, while the fluidity of the movements ensures that grace and poise are never compromised.

3. Tailored to Tackle Female-Specific Concerns:

Issues like osteoporosis, which predominantly affects women, can be countered with weight-bearing exercises. Wall Pilates, with its emphasis on resistance and alignment, is ideal for improving bone density and health.

4. A Safe Space for Expression:

The meditative quality of Wall Pilates offers women a momentary escape. In a world that often demands women to wear multiple hats, this practice becomes a space where they can reconnect with themselves, express their vulnerabilities, and find their inner strength.

5. Aiding Posture and Elegance:

The sedentary lifestyles of today, paired with the commonality of desk jobs, lead to posture issues. For women, who often grapple with the additional weight of breasts, this can lead to severe back and neck problems. Wall Pilates, with its emphasis on spinal alignment and core strength, directly combats these concerns.

6. Empowerment and Confidence:

There's something incredibly empowering about pushing against a wall – a metaphorical challenge – and seeing oneself grow stronger with each session. The confidence gained in a Wall Pilates class extends beyond the studio, enabling women to stand taller in every aspect of their lives.

7. Building Community and Sisterhood:

Women thrive in communities. The shared journey of growth, struggle, and success in a Wall Pilates class fosters deep bonds of sisterhood. Women not only gain a workout partner but often a confidante, a supporter, and a friend.

In conclusion, Wall Pilates isn't just a workout; it's a holistic approach to well-being tailored for the modern woman. It recognizes her struggles, celebrates her strengths, and offers a path that aligns with her unique physical and emotional journey.

Understanding Wall Pilates

A Brief History of Pilates

To fully understand Wall Pilates, it's essential to go back to the roots of Pilates itself. The story of Pilates is as intriguing as the exercises themselves, steeped in history, perseverance, and evolution.

1. The Origin – Joseph Pilates:

Born in 1883 in Germany, Joseph Hubertus Pilates was a sickly child, suffering from asthma, rickets, and rheumatic fever. Determined not to let these ailments define his life, he embarked on a journey to enhance his physical strength. By combining aspects of yoga, martial arts, bodybuilding, and gymnastics, Joseph crafted a unique exercise system.

2. The Early Form – Contrology:

Joseph referred to his method as "Contrology," emphasizing the importance of mind over muscle. It wasn't just about physical strength; it was a holistic approach that combined body and mind. He believed that with the right mental control, the body could be trained to move in any way.

3. Pilates and World War I:

During World War I, Joseph found himself in an internment camp in England. Here, he started refining his techniques, working with other inmates, especially those injured or bedridden. He improvised equipment using springs from hospital beds, laying the groundwork for the specialized Pilates equipment we see today.

4. Moving to America:

In the 1920s, Joseph moved to New York City, where he and his wife Clara opened a fitness studio. Here, they introduced Pilates to dancers, actors, and athletes. The method quickly gained traction, especially in the dance community, due to its emphasis on strength, flexibility, and posture.

5. Legacy and Evolution:

After Joseph's death in 1967, his students, often referred to as the "Elders," continued to teach and propagate his methods. They opened studios, trained new instructors, and ensured that Pilates' teachings lived on. Over the years, as the world changed and new fitness trends emerged, Pilates also evolved. Various branches emerged, each interpreting Joseph's teachings in slightly different ways.

6. The Birth of Wall Pilates:

While traditional Pilates primarily utilized mats and specialized equipment like the Reformer, Cadillac, and Wunda Chair, the 21st century saw the rise of Wall Pilates. By using the wall as resistance, this method combined the core principles of Pilates with the benefits of vertical exercises, offering a fresh take on a century-old practice.

In conclusion, Pilates, from its humble beginnings in a German town to its global recognition today, is a testament to the vision and dedication of Joseph Pilates. It's a reminder that with passion and innovation, any concept can stand the test of time, evolving and adapting to meet the needs of new generations.

Wall Pilates: A Revolution in Fitness

Wall Pilates, while building upon the traditional Pilates foundation, has swiftly become a beacon of innovation in the realm of fitness. This variation, which beautifully fuses the core tenets of Pilates with the unique challenges of utilizing a wall, has breathed fresh life into an already dynamic discipline.
At its core, Pilates is about harmony and balance, not just in our bodies but in our minds. Joseph Pilates crafted a system that integrated physical and mental well-being. And Wall Pilates, while appearing as a departure from the traditional, only amplifies this integration.
Imagine the wall not just as a surface but as an anchor. In Wall Pilates, this anchor becomes an agent of resistance, balance, and support. As participants press against it, stretch alongside it, or use it for balance, the wall becomes a silent partner, challenging them at every step, demanding precision, control, and awareness.
The revolution of Wall Pilates lies in its inclusivity.

Traditional Pilates equipment, while effective, can sometimes be intimidating for beginners. The reformers, chairs, and barrels each have their learning curves. However, a wall is universal. We've all leaned against one, pushed off from one, felt its solid support. Transitioning this everyday experience into a fitness regimen makes Wall Pilates accessible to many who might've hesitated to step into a Pilates studio. Beyond accessibility, Wall Pilates provides a unique set of benefits. The vertical exercises and the act of working against gravity engage muscles differently. There's a heightened awareness of posture when one is upright, leading to a natural focus on alignment. The resistance the wall offers can be as gentle or as challenging as needed, making it adaptable for both novices and seasoned practitioners. This adaptability ensures that every session can be tailored to meet an individual's needs, making progress palpable and, more importantly, achievable.

Moreover, Wall Pilates doesn't just stop at physical transformation. The wall, in many ways, mirrors life's challenges. It's unyielding, solid, and ever-present. As practitioners push against it, finding their rhythm, their strength, and their balance, they're not just building physical resilience. They're learning perseverance, understanding that every challenge, no matter how insurmountable it appears, can be overcome with patience, effort, and a deep connection between mind and body.

In this ever-evolving world of fitness, where trends come and go, Wall Pilates stands out. Not just as a fad, but as a meaningful evolution. It holds onto the heart of what Joseph Pilates envisioned while making it relevant for the modern woman, proving once again that the principles of balance, strength, and mind-body harmony are timeless.

Benefits of Wall Pilates: Beyond Just Toning

In the realm of fitness, it's often easy to get captivated by the allure of visible results. Toned muscles, a sculpted physique, and improved flexibility are undeniably appealing. But Wall Pilates, much like the rest of its Pilates family, offers benefits that go far beyond the mirror's reflection.

Wall Pilates acts as a bridge, connecting our inner and outer worlds. While its physical advantages are undeniable, its more profound impacts lie in the realms of mental, emotional, and holistic health.

A Mental Oasis in a Busy World

The gentle rhythms of Wall Pilates require concentration, pulling us away from the daily bustle and into the present moment. The wall, steadfast and unchanging, reminds us of the importance of grounding ourselves amidst life's chaos. Each movement becomes a meditation, allowing practitioners to cultivate a mental clarity often elusive in our fast-paced lives.

Emotional Resilience through Physical Challenges

Every push against the wall, every stretch, every hold, becomes symbolic of life's adversities. Wall Pilates teaches us persistence. There's an emotional strength that's nurtured as we face, adapt to, and eventually conquer each physical challenge the wall poses. Over time, this resilience built within the confines of a studio starts seeping into everyday life, preparing us for emotional hurdles with a newfound grace.

Deepening Body Awareness and Intuition

Wall Pilates enhances our bodily intuition. As practitioners learn to listen to their body's signals during a workout, they cultivate a heightened sense of what their body needs outside the studio. This intuition helps in making better nutritional choices, understanding the importance of rest, and even in recognizing the first signs of potential health issues.

Harmony and Balance in All Facets

Wall Pilates isn't just about strengthening the body; it's about achieving equilibrium. And this balance isn't limited to physical stability. The holistic approach of Wall Pilates permeates all facets of life. Practitioners often find a more harmonious balance between work and relaxation, between social commitments and solitude, between activity and rest.

Cultivating a Deeper Connection

Lastly, the wall, ever-present and unyielding, becomes more than just an exercise tool. It morphs into a reflection of the world around us, reminding practitioners of the connections we share with our environment. In pushing against the wall, in feeling its support and resistance, there's a silent acknowledgment of our interconnectedness, a subtle nod to the idea that we're all part of something larger.

In essence, Wall Pilates offers a journey, a holistic path that's as much about self-discovery as it is about fitness. It's an invitation to look beyond the superficial and delve deep, to find strength, peace, and balance in both body and spirit.

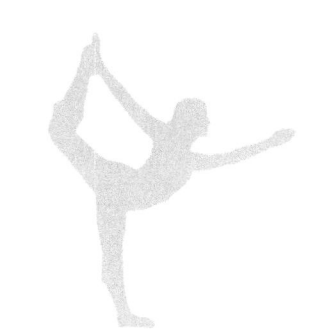

Meet Sarah

Sarah's Journey: A Struggle for Balance and Strength

Sarah always seemed like she had it all together. From the outside, her life appeared picture-perfect: a successful job, a loving family, and weekends filled with laughter and adventure. But underneath that polished exterior, she was waging a silent war with herself.

A Dance of Imbalance

From her early twenties, Sarah faced the constant ebb and flow of weight fluctuations. Every new diet trend became her obsession, from juice cleanses to keto regimes, in hopes of finding that elusive balance. But with each failed attempt, her self-esteem plummeted further, and her body felt like an unfamiliar terrain.

Her career, though flourishing, was demanding. Long hours at the desk, coupled with the pressure to excel, took a toll on her posture. Every night she would return home, her shoulders hunched and back aching, yearning for relief.

Seeking Strength in All the Wrong Places

In her quest for a solution, Sarah tried numerous fitness regimens. High-intensity workouts promised fast results, but they left her feeling drained and, at times, even injured. Yoga offered peace and flexibility, but it couldn't address her specific needs for toning and posture correction.

It was during a weekend retreat with her friends that she first heard about Wall Pilates. Clara, one of the attendees, couldn't stop raving about how it had transformed her life. Initially skeptical, Sarah's curiosity was piqued.

A Doorway to Transformation

Her first Wall Pilates session was nothing short of revelatory. The wall, a seemingly simple prop, challenged her in ways she hadn't anticipated. Every movement was a test of her strength, balance, and coordination. Yet, unlike her past experiences, she didn't feel overwhelmed. Instead, she felt supported and anchored.

Weeks turned into months, and the changes in Sarah became evident. Not just in her toned physique, but in the way she carried herself. The drooping shoulders were now pulled back confidently. The constant backaches became a thing of the past.

More than the physical changes, Wall Pilates gifted Sarah a new perspective. She learned the value of patience, understanding that transformation doesn't happen overnight. She found strength in vulnerability, realizing it's okay to lean on something or someone, much like how she leaned on the wall during her exercises.

A Beacon for Others

Sarah's journey is a testament to the transformative power of Wall Pilates. It's not just about toning muscles or correcting posture. It's about rediscovering oneself, understanding one's limits, and pushing boundaries. It's about finding balance in life, both literally and metaphorically.

Sarah became a beacon of hope for many. Her story inspired countless women who, like her, were on a quest for balance and strength. Through her journey, they saw a reflection of their struggles and, more importantly, a glimpse of the potential that Wall Pilates held for them.

The Science Behind Sarah's Needs and How Wall Pilates Can Address Them

Sarah's journey, like many women's, is a blend of physical and emotional challenges. These challenges arise from various factors, including biology, lifestyle, and the societal pressures women face daily. To genuinely understand how Wall Pilates became a game-changer for her, it's crucial to delve into the science behind her needs.

The Physiology of Posture and Balance

Human posture is dictated by a complex interplay of muscles, bones, and the nervous system. A sedentary lifestyle, which includes prolonged periods of sitting, weakens the core muscles responsible for maintaining an upright position. The spine, designed to bear the body's weight efficiently, starts compensating for this weakened core, leading to imbalances and, eventually, chronic pain.

Balance, on the other hand, is controlled by the vestibular system in our inner ear, our eyes, and proprioceptors in our muscles and joints. As we age or lead a sedentary lifestyle, these systems' efficiency diminishes, increasing the risk of falls and injuries.

Emotional Well-being and Body Image

Beyond the physical, the psychological aspect of body image plays a profound role in a woman's well-being. The societal obsession with an 'ideal' body type can lead to a continuous cycle of diets and rigorous exercise regimens, often at the expense of health. This continuous pursuit can result in a negative self-image, anxiety, and even depression.

How Wall Pilates Comes into Play

Wall Pilates, at its core, is a holistic exercise that aims to restore the body's natural balance. Using the wall as a prop offers resistance, allowing for the activation and strengthening of core muscles. This resistance training, combined with the stretching exercises of Pilates, provides an integrated solution for posture correction and muscle toning.

But the benefits of Wall Pilates go beyond the physical. The focus on controlled movements and breathing creates a meditative space, offering a reprieve from the stresses of daily life. The wall, while initially a tool for exercises, becomes a symbol of support, reminding practitioners like Sarah that leaning on something doesn't signify weakness but is, in fact, a strength.

Furthermore, the systematic progression of exercises in Wall Pilates ensures that every individual works at their pace. This approach fosters a positive relationship with one's body, shifting the focus from societal standards of beauty to personal well-being and strength.

In addressing Sarah's needs, Wall Pilates did more than just tone her muscles or improve her posture. It offered her a sanctuary—a space where she could connect with her body, understand its needs, and work towards fulfilling them, all while being grounded in scientific principles that prioritize holistic health and well-being.

Emotions, Physical Health, and Wall Pilates

In the bustling rhythm of modern life, where the lines between emotional and physical well-being are increasingly blurred, many women like Sarah seek sanctuary. They yearn for a space that allows them to reconnect, not only with their bodies but also with their emotional selves. Wall Pilates emerges as a bridge between these two worlds, interweaving the realms of emotions and physical health.

The Body-Mind Connection

It's a known fact that our emotions and physical health are intrinsically linked. The stress of a demanding job or personal pressures can manifest as tension in the neck, back pain, or even digestive issues. Conversely, persistent physical ailments can lead to feelings of anxiety, depression, or lowered self-esteem. The body and mind, in their innate wisdom, speak to each other, reflecting and responding to every ebb and flow of our emotional state.

Wall Pilates: A Dance of Emotion and Motion

Wall Pilates isn't just an exercise—it's a symphony of movement and emotion. Every stretch, every controlled motion brings forth not just a physical response but an emotional one. As Sarah pushes against the wall, she's not just engaging her muscles; she's also pushing against the weight of her insecurities, her fears, and her challenges. The wall becomes a canvas where she paints her story, one stretch at a time.

The deliberate focus on breathing, a core element of Wall Pilates, amplifies this emotional release. As breath flows, it carries with it the burdens of the heart, making room for clarity, peace, and self-love. Each inhalation draws in hope, and every exhalation releases the chains of past regrets and future anxieties.

A Sanctuary of Self-Discovery

For Sarah and countless other women, Wall Pilates transforms into a journey of self-discovery. In the quiet moments, when she's holding a pose against the wall, she confronts her vulnerabilities. She meets her strengths, acknowledges her weaknesses, and embraces the entirety of her being. The wall, steadfast and supportive, reflects back to her a narrative of resilience, empowerment, and grace.

In the dance of Wall Pilates, emotions and physical health waltz in harmony. It's a reminder that healing isn't just about toned muscles or perfect posture; it's about mending the heart, quieting the mind, and celebrating the beautiful, intricate tapestry of our human experience.

Starting Your Wall Pilates Routine

Preparing Your Space: Safety First

The tranquility and focus of Wall Pilates can only be truly harnessed when one's environment is both physically safe and emotionally inviting. As with any fitness routine, the first step isn't the exercise itself, but rather preparing a conducive environment. But Wall Pilates, being such a unique blend of motion and emotion, requires a touch more foresight.

The Sanctity of Your Space

When we talk about 'space' in Wall Pilates, it isn't just the physical dimensions we refer to, but the ambiance and energy as well. Your space should resonate with calmness, inviting your mind to release its clutter and your body to move freely. Think of it as creating a mini sanctuary where the outside world momentarily fades, allowing you to center yourself.

Sturdy Walls, Sturdy Foundations

While the ambiance is essential, the physical robustness of your wall cannot be overlooked. It should be free from obstructions like paintings, shelves, or any decor. Ensure the wall you choose is sturdy, offering robust support. The last thing you'd want is to second guess the wall's reliability mid-exercise.

Floor Matters

While Wall Pilates focuses primarily on the wall, let's not forget the importance of the floor. A non-slippery surface ensures safety during movements that require you to be both on the floor and against the wall. Whether it's hardwood, carpet, or tiles, ensure you have a good-quality mat to provide cushioning and prevent slipping.

Ventilation and Lighting

Breathing is a central tenet of Wall Pilates. It stands to reason then that your space should be well-ventilated. Fresh air not only aids in better respiratory function but also invigorates the senses, enhancing your workout experience. Equally important is lighting.

Soft, natural light can be invigorating and soothing, setting the tone for your Wall Pilates session.

Final Touches

Lastly, consider adding personal touches. Maybe it's a scented candle whose aroma calms your mind, or perhaps it's a plant that adds a touch of nature to your indoor space. Whatever you choose, let it resonate with your spirit, turning your Wall Pilates corner into a personal haven.

In preparing your space, you're not just setting the stage for a workout but signaling to your mind and body that this is a sacred time. A time of self-care, introspection, and growth. Safety might be the primary objective, but in the process, you're also creating a cocoon of serenity and strength.

The Basic Gear: From Mats to Grip Socks

Stepping into the world of Wall Pilates is akin to embracing a dance of grace, balance, and strength. But like any art form or discipline, having the right tools can transform one's experience from mediocre to extraordinary. While the essence of Wall Pilates lies in the flow of movement and the core principles guiding each pose, the importance of the right gear can't be understated.

The Foundation: Your Mat

Think of your mat as the canvas upon which your Wall Pilates journey unfolds. It's not just about cushioning against the hard floor, but about providing a tactile feedback loop as you shift your weight, balance, and align your body. The right mat complements your movements, offering just enough grip without being sticky, and enough cushion without being overly soft. It becomes an extension of you, grounding you as you reach, stretch, and push against the wall.

Grip Socks: Your Silent Partners

Then come the grip socks, those unsung heroes in your Wall Pilates journey. These aren't ordinary socks; they're designed with purpose. Their grip pattern is crafted to provide stability even in the most challenging poses, ensuring that your feet, often the primary points of contact with the ground, are stable and supported. But it's not just about physical grip. The confidence these socks imbue, the assurance that you won't slip, allows you to immerse deeper into each movement, fully present and engaged.

Comfort Meets Function: Appropriate Attire

While Wall Pilates doesn't demand a specific uniform, what you wear significantly impacts your experience. The ideal attire marries comfort with function. You need clothing that moves with you, not against you. Fabrics that breathe, allowing your skin to feel cool even as your body heats up. Yet, they should be form-fitting enough so that they don't get in your way or become a distraction.

Accessories with Purpose

While the mat and socks are the primary gear pieces, don't overlook the potential accessories that might enhance your Wall Pilates sessions. Perhaps it's a soft headband that keeps sweat and hair away from your eyes, or a subtle wristband that offers support during certain poses. These items, while not essential, can add that touch of personalization and functionality to your routine.

In Wall Pilates, as in life, sometimes it's the seemingly small things that make a significant difference. It's not about amassing a collection of gear but about finding those few, well-chosen pieces that elevate your practice. In doing so, you not only ensure safety and functionality but also infuse a touch of your personality into your Wall Pilates journey, making it uniquely and beautifully yours.

🎁Get your gift🎁

Scan this QR code

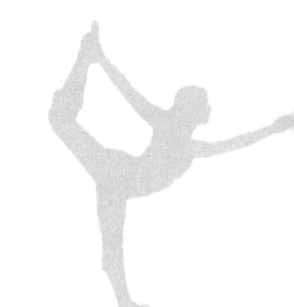

Beginner Wall Pilates Exercises

Wall Roll-Up: Duration: 1 minute Repetitions: 10 times

1. Position: Begin standing with your back against the wall. Your feet should be hip-width apart and a foot away from the wall. Extend your arms in front of you.

2. Movement: Inhale deeply. As you exhale, tuck your chin to your chest and start to roll down vertebra by vertebra, keeping your hands parallel to the floor. Inhale at the bottom of the movement. Exhale and reverse, rolling up and stacking each vertebra, returning to the starting position.

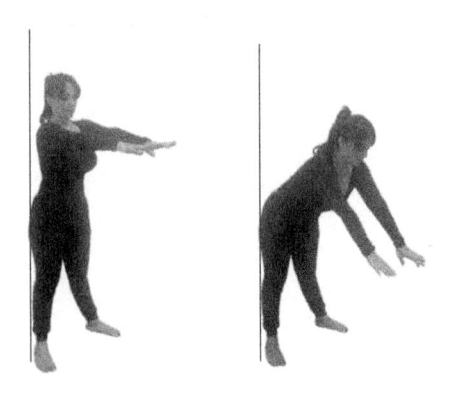

Wall Saw: Duration:

1 minute Repetitions: 10 times per side

1. Position: Stand with your back against the wall and spread your feet wider than hip-width. Stretch your arms out to the sides, in line with your shoulders.

2. Movement: Inhale deeply. Exhale and twist your torso to the right, reaching your left hand towards your right foot. Inhale to return to the center. Repeat on the other side.

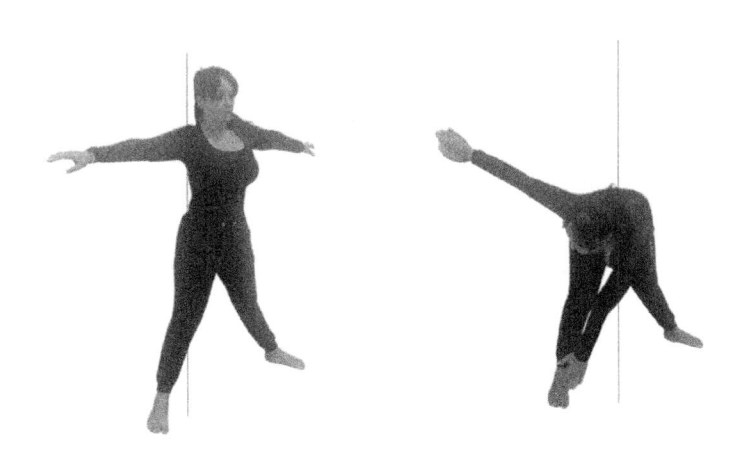

Wall Plank and Push-Up

Duration: 2 minutes Repetitions: 15 push-ups

1. Position: Begin in a plank position with your hands against the wall, directly below your shoulders.

2. Movement: Inhale as you bend your elbows, bringing your chest closer to the wall. Exhale, pushing through your palms, and extend your arms back to the plank position.

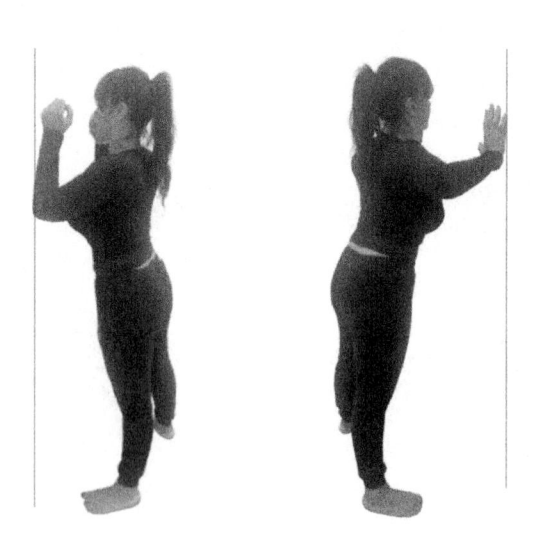

Wall Pelvic Curl: Duration: 1 minute Repetitions: 12 times

1. Position: Lie on the floor with your feet flat on the wall, knees bent at a 90-degree angle.

2. Movement: Inhale deeply. As you exhale, press into your feet and peel your spine off the ground, starting with your tailbone and moving up vertebra by vertebra. Inhale at the top and exhale as you lower down, articulating your spine onto the floor.

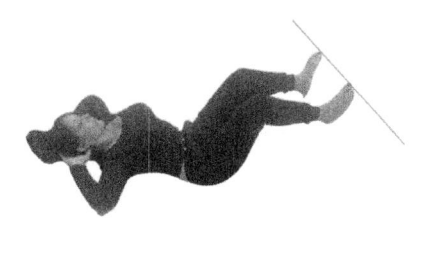

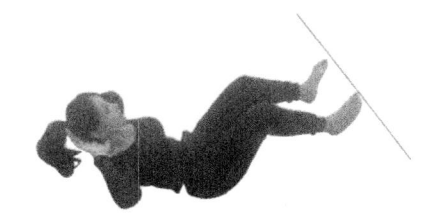

Wall Chest Lift:

Duration: 1 minute Repetitions: 12 times

1. Position: Lie on the ground with your knees bent and feet on the wall. Place your hands behind your head.

2. Movement: Inhale deeply. As you exhale, engage your core and lift your head and upper back off the floor. Inhale to lower back down.

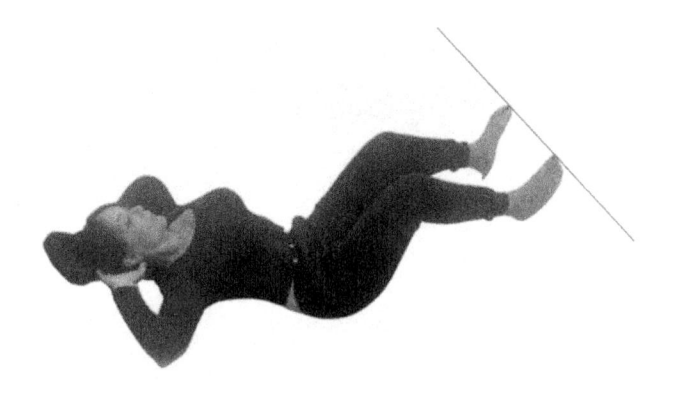

Standing Leg Lift:

Duration: 2 minutes (1 minute per side) Repetitions: 15 times per side

1. Position: Stand tall with your right side against the wall, right hand resting on it for balance.

2. Movement: Engage your core and lift your left leg out to the side as high as comfortable. Lower down with control.

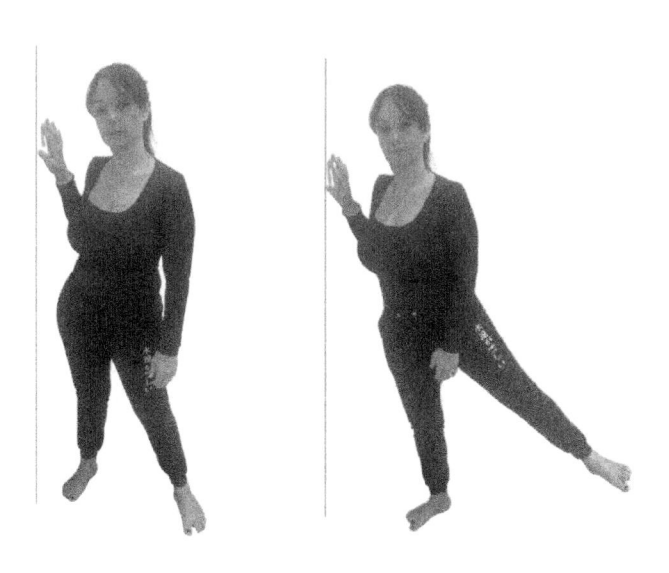

Wall Side Kick Series:

Duration: 2 minutes (1 minute per side) Repetitions: 12 swings per side

1. Position: Stand with your right side against the wall, right hand resting on it for balance.

2. Movement: Engage your core and extend your left leg straight in front of you. Swing the leg back, then return it to the front in a controlled motion.

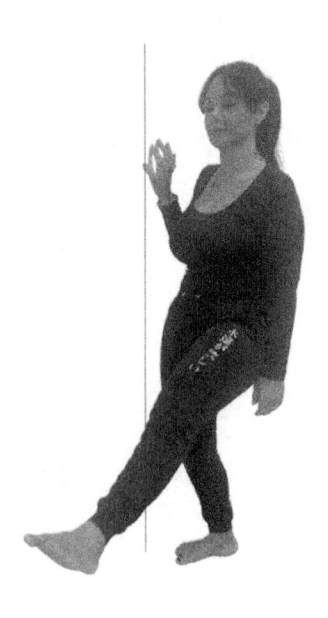

Wall Spine Twist:

Duration: 1 minute Repetitions: 10 times per side

1. Position: Sit on the floor with your back against the wall, legs extended in front of you.

2. Movement: Inhale deeply. Exhale and twist your torso to the right, reaching your left hand towards your right foot. Return to center and repeat on the opposite side.

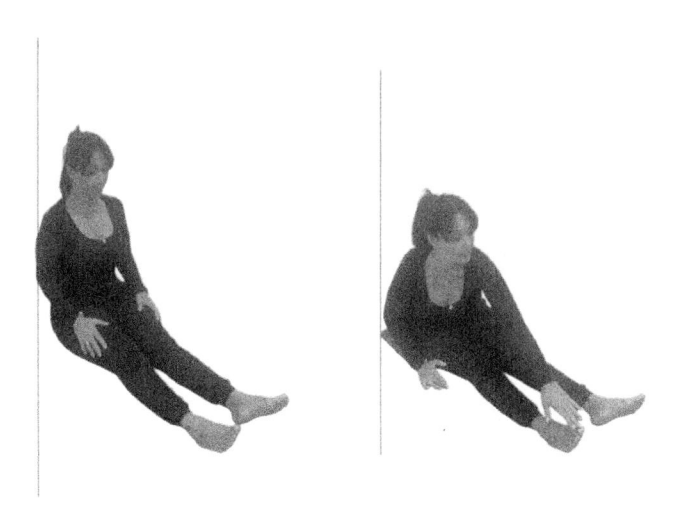

Arm Circles Against Wall:

Duration: 1 minute Repetitions: 10 circles in each direction

1. Position: Stand facing the wall with arms extended in front of you, hands flat on the wall.

2. Movement: Circle your arms up, out to the sides, and then down, keeping hands in contact with the wall. Imagine tracing a large circle with your fingertips while your hands remain in contact with the wall.

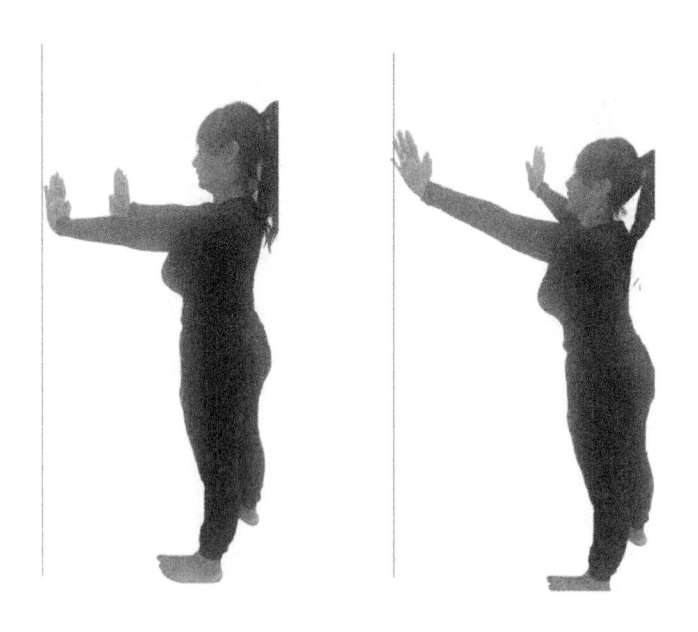

Wall Leg Slides:

Duration: 2 minutes Repetitions: 10 times per leg

1. Position: Lie on the floor with your legs straight up against the wall, bottoms of the feet touching the wall.

2. Movement: Engage your core and slide one leg down the wall while keeping the other leg stable. Slide the leg back up and switch sides.

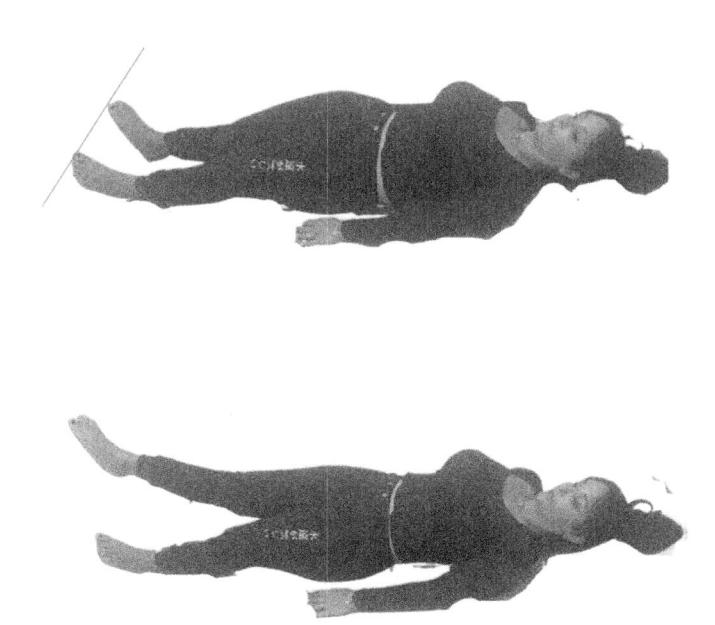

Wall Climbing Series:

Duration: 1 minute Repetitions: 10 climbs up and down

1. Position: Stand facing the wall, place your hands flat on the wall at chest height.

2. Movement: Begin to walk your hands up the wall as you lean in, then walk them back down to the starting position.

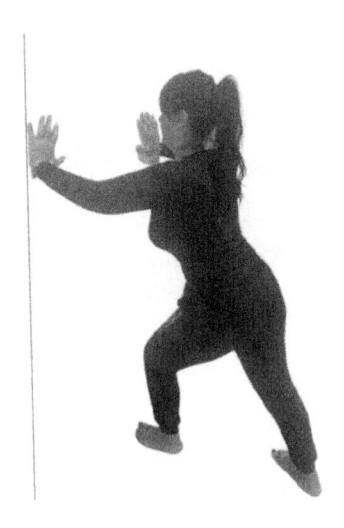

Remember, it's essential to maintain proper form throughout each exercise to maximize benefits and prevent injury.

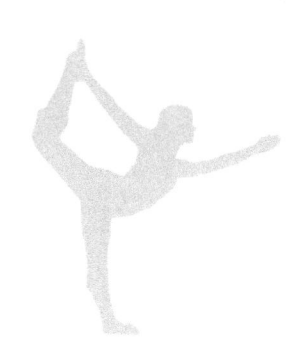

Intermediate Wall Pilates Techniques

Wall Supported Bridge:

Duration: 1.5 minutes Repetitions: 12 times

1. Position: Lie on the floor with your knees bent and feet flat against the wall. Arms rest by your sides.

2. Movement: Push through the feet and lift the hips off the ground, forming a straight line from shoulders to knees. Hold the top position briefly before slowly lowering your spine back to the floor.

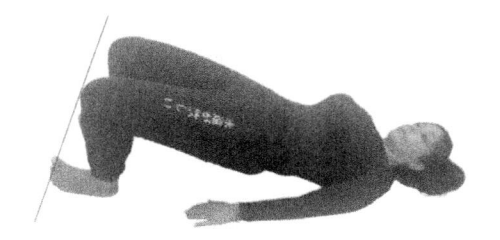

Wall Ballet Stretches:

Duration: 2 minutes (1 minute per leg)
Repetitions: Hold each stretch for 30 seconds, switch legs and repeat.

1. Position: Stand tall facing the wall with your arms stretched out and hands pressed against the wall for support.

2. Movement: Lift one leg and place the ankle or calf against the wall, keeping the other leg straight. Gently press into the wall to deepen the stretch. Switch legs.

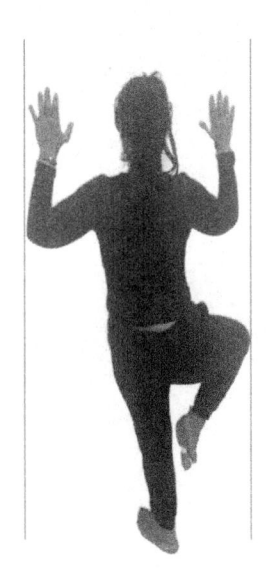

Extended Wall Leg Stretch:

Duration: 2 minutes (1 minute per leg)
Repetitions: Hold each stretch for 30 seconds, switch legs and repeat.

1. Position: Sit down with one side against the wall, extending the leg that's closest to the wall straight up.

2. Movement: Gently pull the elevated leg towards you, deepening the stretch, while the other leg remains extended on the floor.

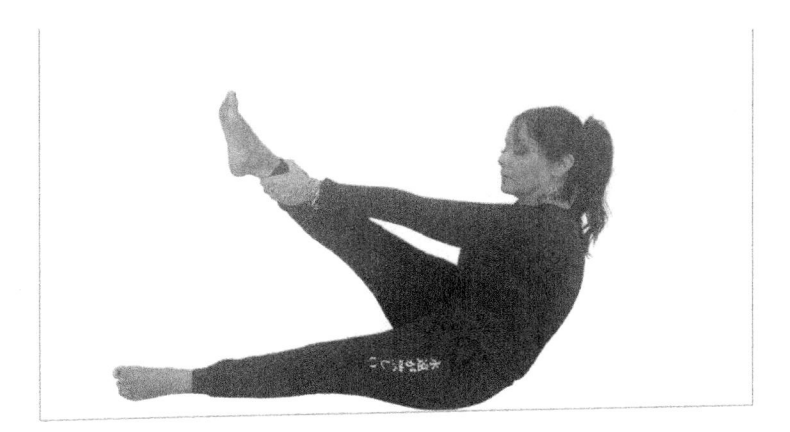

Wall Scissors:

Duration: 2 minutes Repetitions: 15 times per leg

1. Position: Lie on the floor, legs straight up against the wall, and arms resting by your sides.

2. Movement: Lower one leg down toward the ground while keeping the other against the wall. Alternate legs in a scissor-like motion.

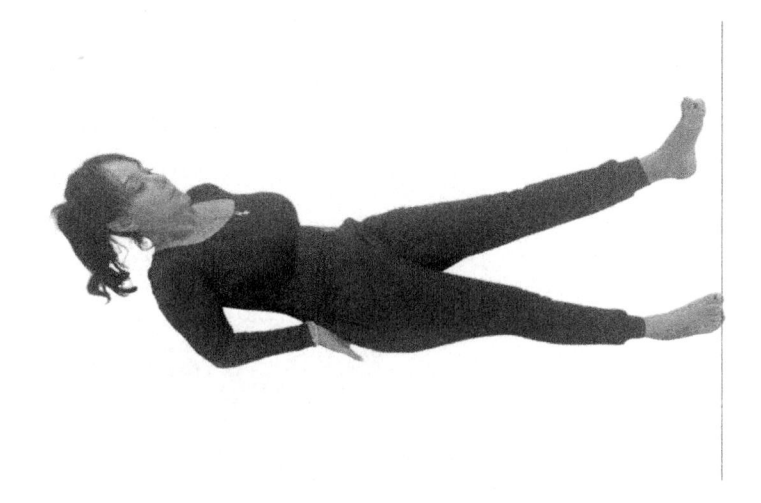

Wall Side Plank Series:

Duration: 2 minutes (1 minute per side)

Repetitions: 10 lifts and lowers per side

1. Position: Begin in a side plank position with your lower hand against the wall for support and upper arm extended towards the ceiling.

2. Movement: Lift and lower your hips, maintaining a straight line from head to heels.

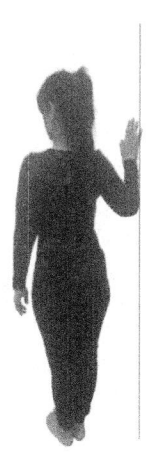

Wall Teaser Prep:

Duration: 1.5 minutes Repetitions: 10 times

1. Position: Sit on the floor with your knees bent and feet on the wall.

2. Movement: Lean back, balancing on your sit bones while extending your arms parallel to the floor. Hold, then return to the starting position.

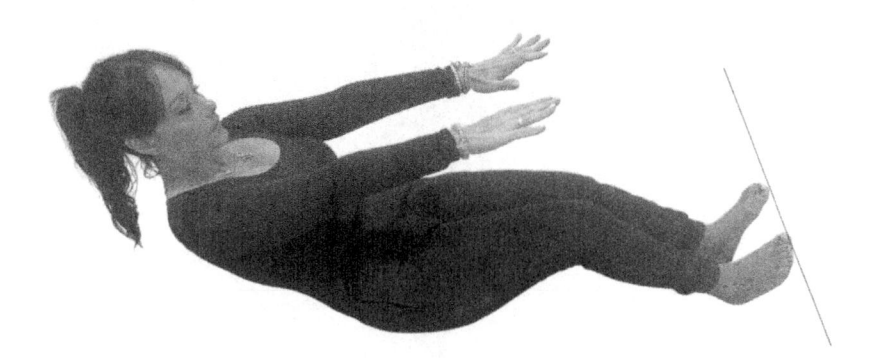

Wall Leg Circles:

Duration: 2.5 minutes (1.25 minutes per leg)
Repetitions: 10 circles in each direction per leg

1. Position: Lie on the floor beside the wall, one leg extended upwards on the wall and the other flat on the floor.

2. Movement: Circle the elevated leg in controlled motions without moving the pelvis.

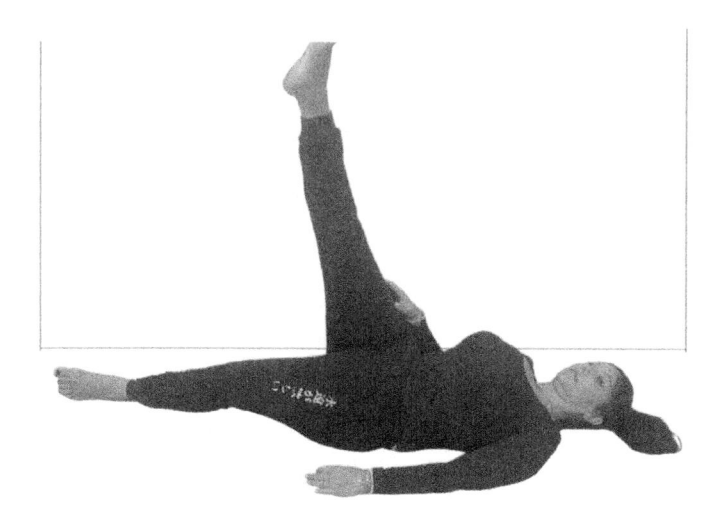

Wall Swan Dive:

Duration: 1 minute Repetitions: 10 times

1. Position: Stand facing away from the wall with your hands against it, arms fully extended and feet hip-width apart.

2. Movement: Engage your core and bend backward, creating an arch with your back, then return to the starting position.

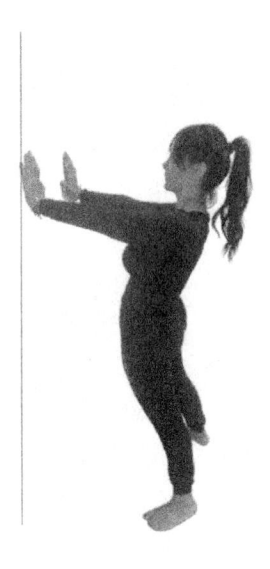

Wall Lateral Flexion:

Duration: 2 minutes (1 minute per side)
Repetitions: 10 times per side

1. Position: Stand with your right side against the wall and left arm extended overhead.

2. Movement: Bend to the left, sliding your hand down your side, then return to the starting position. Switch sides.

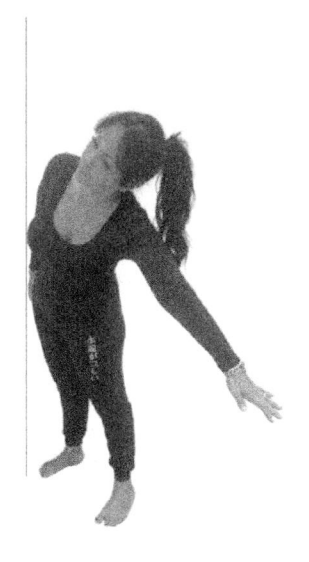

Wall Hip Stretch:

Duration: 2 minutes (1 minute per leg)
Repetitions: Hold each stretch for 30 seconds, switch legs and repeat.

1. Position: Stand facing the wall with one foot resting on the wall at hip level.

2. Movement: Gently press forward, feeling a stretch in the front of the hip of the elevated leg.

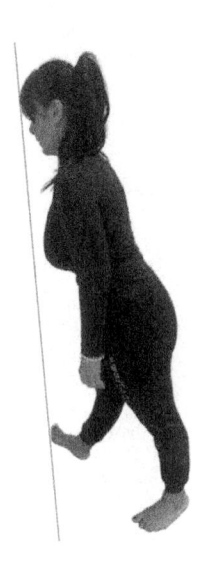

Wall Oblique Roll-Up:

Duration: 2 minutes (1 minute per side)
Repetitions: 10 times per side

1. Position: Lie on the floor with your left side facing the wall, legs slightly forward and hands behind your head.

2. Movement: Engage your obliques and lift your torso off the ground, aiming to touch the wall. Lower down and repeat on the other side.

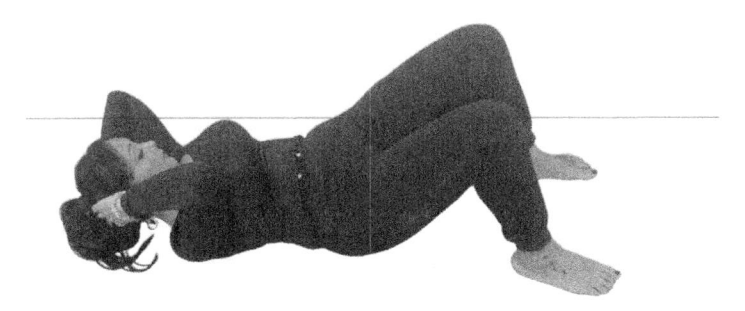

Always ensure you maintain proper form during these exercises to maximize benefits and prevent potential injury.

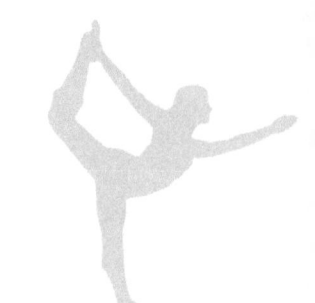

Advanced Wall Pilates Exercises

Wall Jack Knife:

Duration: 2,5 minutes Repetitions: 15 times

1. Position: Start lying down on the floor with legs extended upwards against the wall and arms by your sides.

2. Movement: Engage your core and lift your hips off the ground, pushing your legs towards the ceiling. Slowly lower back down with control.

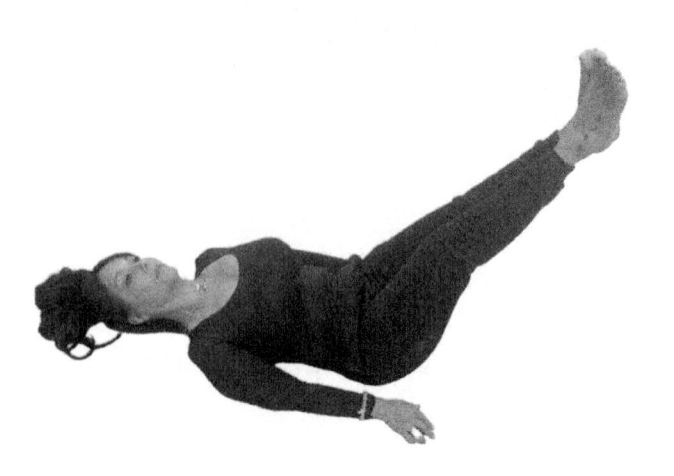

Wall Twist:

Duration: 2 minutes (1 minute per side)
Repetitions: 15 times per side

1. Position: Sit with your left hip against the wall, feet flat on the floor, and hands behind your head.

2. Movement: Rotate your torso to the right, aiming to touch the wall with your left elbow. Return to center and switch sides.

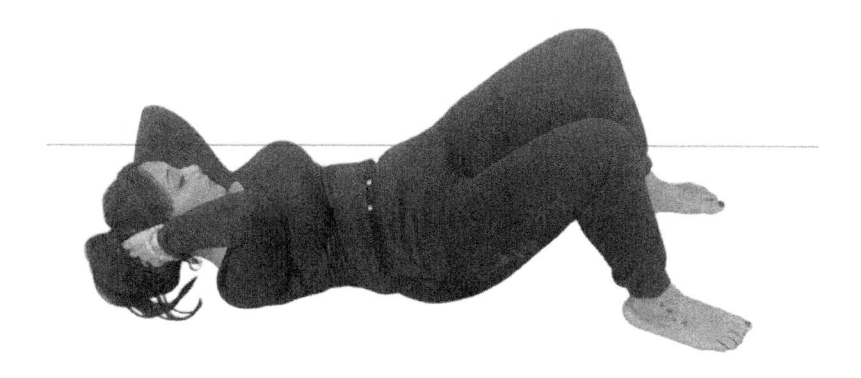

Wall Side Bends:

Duration: 2 minutes (1 minute per side)
Repetitions: 15 times per side

1. Position: Stand with your left side against the wall, feet together, and right arm overhead.

2. Movement: Bend to the right, sliding your right hand down the wall while reaching the left arm overhead. Return to start and switch sides.

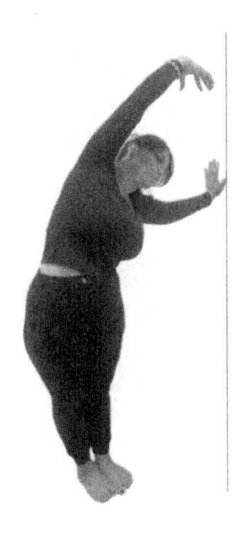

Wall Control Balance:

Duration: 2 minutes

Repetitions: Alternate legs 20 times in total (10 times each leg)

1. Position: Sit on the floor facing the wall, knees bent, and feet pressed against the wall.

2. Movement: Lean back, lifting both feet off the floor, and balance on your sit bones. Extend one leg at a time, pressing the foot against the wall, alternating legs.

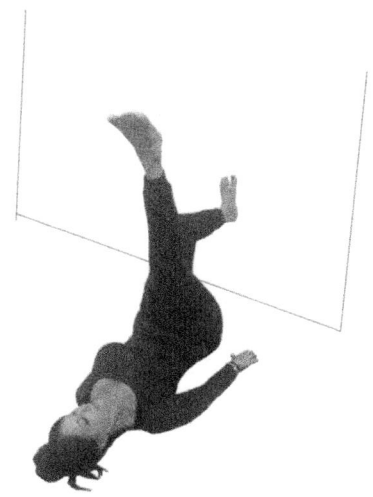

Wall Splits:

Duration: 3 minutes (1.5 minutes per leg)
Repetitions: Hold each stretch for 45 seconds, switch legs, and repeat.

1. Position: Face the wall, placing one foot against it while the other foot is flat on the floor behind you.

2. Movement: Gently press into the wall, extending the front leg and sinking into the stretch. Switch legs.

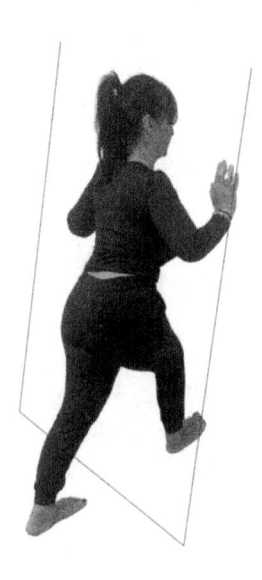

High Intensity Wall Climbs:

Duration: 3 minutes
Repetitions: 12 times up and down the wall

1. Position: Start in a plank position with feet against the wall.

2. Movement: Walk your feet up the wall while keeping the body straight, pushing through your hands and moving one foot at a time, then walk them back down.

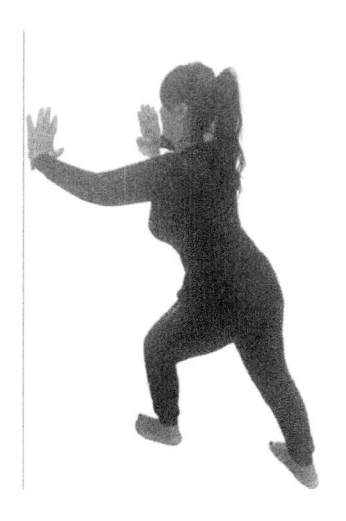

Wall Open Leg Rocker:

Duration: 2 minutes
Repetitions: Rock back and forth 12 times

1. Position: Sit on the floor with legs extended and open in a V-shape, feet pressed against the wall.

2. Movement: Lean back slightly, balance on sit bones, and use your hands to grip the ankles. Rock back and forth while maintaining this position.

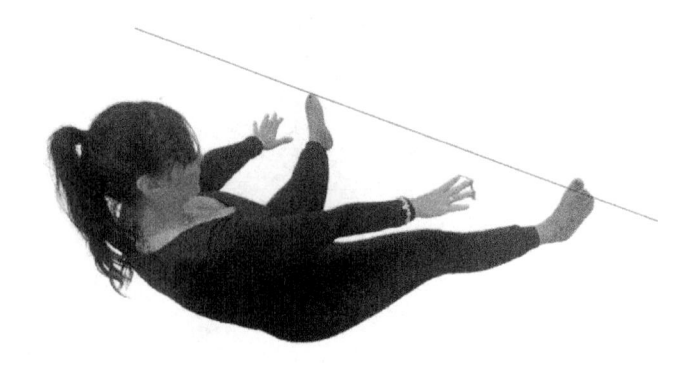

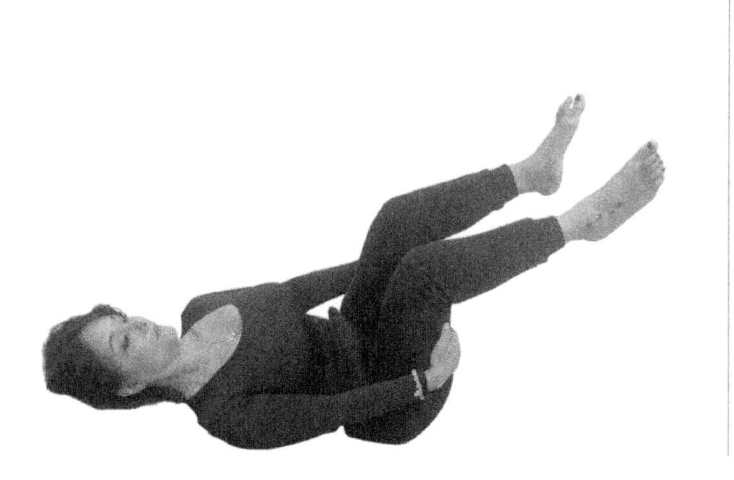

Wall Double Leg Stretch:

Duration: 2 minutes Repetitions: 15 times

1. Position: Lie on the floor, legs extended upwards against the wall, hands on the back of your thighs.

2. Movement: Pull both knees to your chest, then extend them back up the wall.

Wall Single Leg Stretch:

Duration: 2.5 minutes

Repetitions: Alternate legs 20 times in total (10 times each leg)

1. Position: Lie on the floor with one leg extended upwards on the wall and the other knee pulled to your chest.

2. Movement: Alternate legs, pulling one knee to the chest while extending the other up the wall.

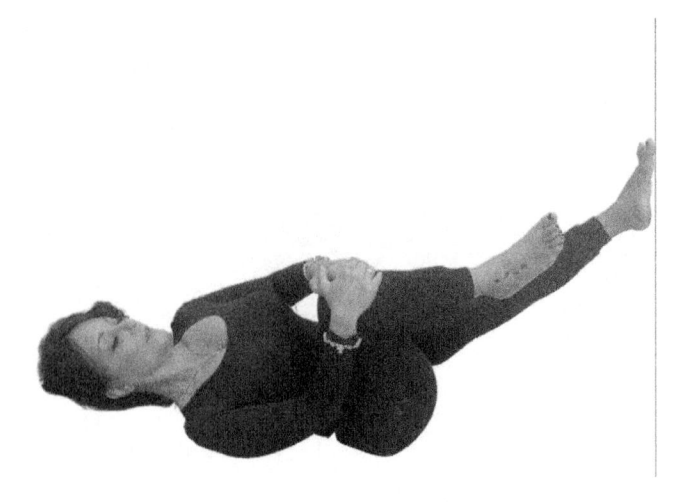

Wall Criss-Cross:

Duration: 2 minutes
Repetitions: 20 times (10 times for each side)

1. Position: Lie on the floor with knees bent, feet on the wall, hands behind the head.

2. Movement: Lift the head and shoulders off the ground, rotate the torso to bring the right elbow towards the left knee, then alternate sides.

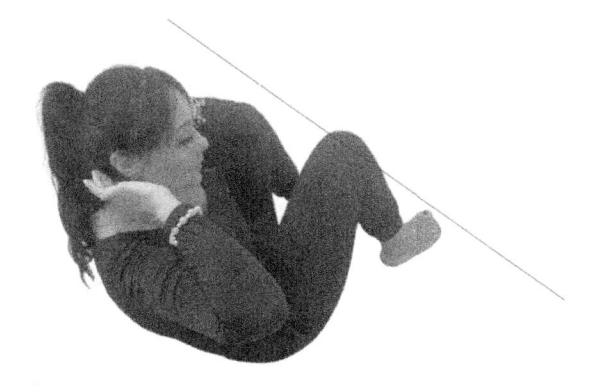

Wall Rollover with Flexion:

Duration: 2,5 minutes Repetitions: 15 times

1. Position: Lie on the floor with legs extended up the wall.

2. Movement: Lift the hips and roll over, bringing the feet towards the floor behind your head. Then, flex the spine to roll back down with control.

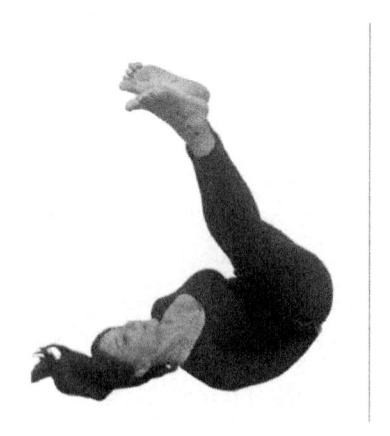

Wall Spine Stretch Forward:

Duration: 1.5 minutes

Repetitions: 10 times, holding each stretch for 3-5 seconds.

1. Position: Sit up tall, legs open wide, feet pressed against the wall.

2. Movement: Hinge forward at the hips, reaching the hands towards the wall while keeping the spine elongated.

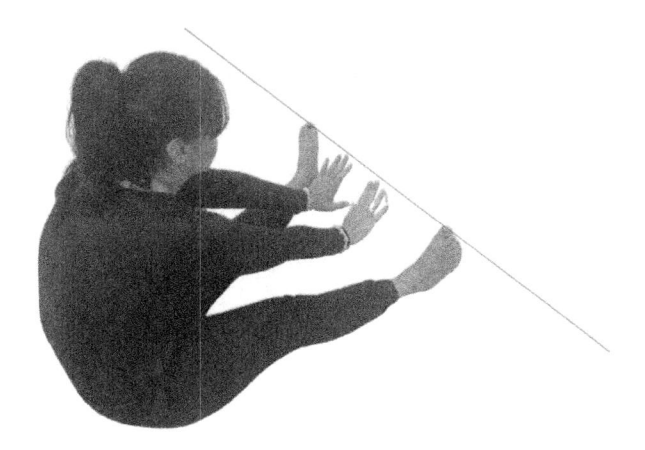

Remember that advanced Pilates exercises require a significant amount of strength, flexibility, and balance. It's crucial to ensure proper technique to avoid injuries. If you're unsure about any movement, it's recommended to consult with a certified Pilates instructor.

🎁 DIGITAL ACCESS 🎁

Scan this QR code

🎁 30-Day Challenge Planner 🎁

If you've been out of the exercise routine for a while and experience fatigue or discomfort post-workout, consider performing these exercises every alternate day for about 5-10 days. This gives your body the chance to adjust to the new movements. Once acclimated, you can then embark on the 30-day challenge.

10-Day Beginner Wall Pilates Workout Plan

Day 1 - Introduction to Wall Pilates:
- Wall Roll-Up: 5 repetitions
- Wall Saw: 5 repetitions
- Wall Plank and Push-Up: 3 repetitions
- Wall Pelvic Curl: 5 repetitions
- Standing Leg Lift: 5 repetitions each leg
- Wall Leg Slides: 5 repetitions

Day 2 - Finding Your Balance:
- Wall Roll-Up: 6 repetitions
- Wall Chest Lift: 5 repetitions
- Wall Plank and Push-Up: 4 repetitions
- Arm Circles Against Wall: 5 repetitions each direction
- Standing Leg Lift: 6 repetitions each leg
- Wall Side Kick Series: 4 repetitions each side

Day 3 - Core Engagement:
- Wall Roll-Up: 7 repetitions
- Wall Saw: 6 repetitions
- Wall Chest Lift: 6 repetitions
- Wall Pelvic Curl: 6 repetitions
- Wall Spine Twist: 5 repetitions each side
- Wall Leg Slides: 6 repetitions

Day 4 - Increasing Strength:
- Wall Roll-Up: 8 repetitions
- Wall Plank and Push-Up: 5 repetitions
- Wall Pelvic Curl: 7 repetitions
- Standing Leg Lift: 7 repetitions each leg
- Arm Circles Against Wall: 6 repetitions each direction
- Wall Climbing Series: 4 repetitions

Day 5 - Challenge Yourself:
- Wall Roll-Up: 9 repetitions
- Wall Saw: 7 repetitions
- Wall Plank and Push-Up: 6 repetitions
- Wall Spine Twist: 6 repetitions each side
- Wall Side Kick Series: 5 repetitions each side
- Wall Leg Slides: 7 repetitions

Day 6 - Halfway through the Basics:
- Wall Roll-Up: 10 repetitions
- Wall Chest Lift: 7 repetitions
- Wall Plank and Push-Up: 7 repetitions
- Standing Leg Lift: 8 repetitions each leg
- Wall Pelvic Curl: 8 repetitions
- Arm Circles Against Wall: 7 repetitions each direction

Day 7 - Push the Limits:
- Wall Roll-Up: 10 repetitions
- Wall Saw: 8 repetitions
- Wall Plank and Push-Up: 8 repetitions
- Wall Spine Twist: 7 repetitions each side
- Wall Side Kick Series: 6 repetitions each side
- Wall Climbing Series: 5 repetitions

Day 8 - Refining the Techniques:
- Wall Roll-Up: 11 repetitions
- Wall Chest Lift: 8 repetitions
- Standing Leg Lift: 9 repetitions each leg
- Wall Pelvic Curl: 9 repetitions
- Wall Leg Slides: 8 repetitions
- Arm Circles Against Wall: 8 repetitions each direction

Day 9 - Strengthen and Lengthen:
- Wall Roll-Up: 12 repetitions
- Wall Plank and Push-Up: 9 repetitions
- Wall Saw: 9 repetitions
- Wall Spine Twist: 8 repetitions each side
- Standing Leg Lift: 10 repetitions each leg
- Wall Climbing Series: 6 repetitions

Day 10 - Building a Strong Foundation:
- Wall Roll-Up: 12 repetitions
- Wall Chest Lift: 9 repetitions
- Wall Plank and Push-Up: 10 repetitions
- Wall Pelvic Curl: 10 repetitions
- Wall Side Kick Series: 7 repetitions each side
- Arm Circles Against Wall: 9 repetitions each direction

Remember, the goal during these 10 days is to familiarize yourself with each exercise and gradually build endurance. Listen to your body and adjust as needed. If an exercise feels too challenging, it's okay to decrease the repetitions or skip it altogether. The key is consistency and progress over perfection.

10-Day Intermediate Wall Pilates Workout Plan

Day 11 - Transitioning to Intermediate:
- Wall Supported Bridge: 5 repetitions
- Wall Ballet Stretches: 5 repetitions each side
- Extended Wall Leg Stretch: 5 repetitions each leg
- Wall Scissors: 6 repetitions
- Wall Side Plank Series: 3 repetitions each side
- Wall Leg Circles: 5 repetitions each direction

Day 12 - Focusing on Flexibility:
- Wall Supported Bridge: 6 repetitions
- Wall Ballet Stretches: 6 repetitions each side
- Wall Hip Stretch: 5 repetitions each side
- Wall Scissors: 7 repetitions
- Wall Teaser Prep: 5 repetitions
- Wall Leg Circles: 6 repetitions each direction

Day 13 - Core Activation:
- Wall Supported Bridge: 7 repetitions
- Wall Ballet Stretches: 7 repetitions each side
- Extended Wall Leg Stretch: 6 repetitions each leg
- Wall Lateral Flexion: 5 repetitions each side
- Wall Side Plank Series: 4 repetitions each side
- Wall Teaser Prep: 6 repetitions

Day 14 - Building on Strength:
- Wall Supported Bridge: 8 repetitions
- Wall Scissors: 8 repetitions
- Wall Ballet Stretches: 8 repetitions each side
- Wall Hip Stretch: 6 repetitions each side
- Wall Oblique Roll-Up: 5 repetitions
- Wall Leg Circles: 7 repetitions each direction

Day 15 - Challenging the Core:
- Wall Supported Bridge: 9 repetitions
- Extended Wall Leg Stretch: 7 repetitions each leg
- Wall Scissors: 9 repetitions
- Wall Side Plank Series: 5 repetitions each side
- Wall Lateral Flexion: 6 repetitions each side
- Wall Teaser Prep: 7 repetitions

Day 16 - Elevating the Intensity:
- Wall Supported Bridge: 10 repetitions
- Wall Ballet Stretches: 9 repetitions each side
- Wall Hip Stretch: 7 repetitions each side
- Wall Scissors: 10 repetitions
- Wall Oblique Roll-Up: 6 repetitions
- Wall Side Plank Series: 6 repetitions each side

Day 17 - Enhancing Flexibility and Strength:
- Wall Supported Bridge: 10 repetitions
- Wall Ballet Stretches: 10 repetitions each side
- Extended Wall Leg Stretch: 8 repetitions each leg
- Wall Teaser Prep: 8 repetitions
- Wall Lateral Flexion: 7 repetitions each side
- Wall Leg Circles: 8 repetitions each direction

Day 18 - Building Endurance:
- Wall Supported Bridge: 11 repetitions
- Wall Scissors: 11 repetitions
- Wall Hip Stretch: 8 repetitions each side
- Wall Ballet Stretches: 10 repetitions each side
- Wall Oblique Roll-Up: 7 repetitions
- Wall Side Plank Series: 7 repetitions each side

Day 19 - Fine-Tuning Techniques:
- Wall Supported Bridge: 12 repetitions
- Extended Wall Leg Stretch: 9 repetitions each leg
- Wall Scissors: 12 repetitions
- Wall Lateral Flexion: 8 repetitions each side
- Wall Teaser Prep: 9 repetitions
- Wall Leg Circles: 9 repetitions each direction

Day 20 - Celebrating Intermediate Mastery:
- Wall Supported Bridge: 12 repetitions
- Wall Ballet Stretches: 11 repetitions each side
- Wall Hip Stretch: 9 repetitions each side
- Wall Scissors: 12 repetitions
- Wall Oblique Roll-Up: 8 repetitions
- Wall Side Plank Series: 8 repetitions each side

As you advance through the intermediate days, ensure you maintain proper form and technique. The intermediate level requires greater strength, balance, and flexibility, so always be mindful of your body's limitations. Modify exercises if necessary, and prioritize quality over quantity. Remember, progress is made through consistent practice and gradual advancement.

10-Day Advanced Wall Pilates Workout Plan

Day 21 - Entering the Advanced Realm:
- Wall Jack Knife: 4 repetitions
- Wall Twist: 4 repetitions each side
- Wall Side Bends: 5 repetitions each side
- Wall Control Balance: 3 repetitions each leg
- Wall Splits: 4 repetitions
- High Intensity Wall Climbs: 3 repetitions

Day 22 - Intensity Uptick:
- Wall Jack Knife: 5 repetitions
- Wall Twist: 5 repetitions each side
- Wall Control Balance: 4 repetitions each leg
- Wall Open Leg Rocker: 3 repetitions
- Wall Double Leg Stretch: 4 repetitions
- Wall Single Leg Stretch: 4 repetitions each leg

Day 23 - Challenging Stability:
- Wall Jack Knife: 5 repetitions
- Wall Side Bends: 6 repetitions each side
- Wall Rollover with Flexion: 4 repetitions
- Wall Splits: 5 repetitions
- Wall Criss-Cross: 4 repetitions each side
- High Intensity Wall Climbs: 4 repetitions

Day 24 - Advanced Flow:
- Wall Twist: 6 repetitions each side
- Wall Control Balance: 5 repetitions each leg
- Wall Open Leg Rocker: 4 repetitions
- Wall Double Leg Stretch: 5 repetitions
- Wall Single Leg Stretch: 5 repetitions each leg
- Wall Spine Stretch Forward: 4 repetitions

Day 25 - Engage and Empower:
- Wall Jack Knife: 6 repetitions
- Wall Side Bends: 7 repetitions each side
- Wall Rollover with Flexion: 5 repetitions
- Wall Criss-Cross: 5 repetitions each side
- Wall Splits: 6 repetitions
- High Intensity Wall Climbs: 5 repetitions

Day 26 - Dynamic Movements:
- Wall Twist: 7 repetitions each side
- Wall Control Balance: 6 repetitions each leg
- Wall Open Leg Rocker: 5 repetitions
- Wall Double Leg Stretch: 6 repetitions
- Wall Single Leg Stretch: 6 repetitions each leg
- Wall Spine Stretch Forward: 5 repetitions

Day 27 - Reach Your Peak:
- Wall Jack Knife: 7 repetitions
- Wall Side Bends: 8 repetitions each side
- Wall Rollover with Flexion: 6 repetitions
- Wall Criss-Cross: 6 repetitions each side
- Wall Splits: 7 repetitions
- High Intensity Wall Climbs: 6 repetitions

Day 28 - Masterful Techniques:
- Wall Twist: 8 repetitions each side
- Wall Control Balance: 7 repetitions each leg
- Wall Open Leg Rocker: 6 repetitions
- Wall Double Leg Stretch: 7 repetitions
- Wall Single Leg Stretch: 7 repetitions each leg
- Wall Spine Stretch Forward: 6 repetitions

Day 29 - Near Finish Line Strength:
- Wall Jack Knife: 8 repetitions
- Wall Side Bends: 9 repetitions each side
- Wall Rollover with Flexion: 7 repetitions
- Wall Criss-Cross: 7 repetitions each side
- Wall Splits: 8 repetitions
- High Intensity Wall Climbs: 7 repetitions

Day 30 - Celebrate Advanced Mastery:
- Wall Twist: 9 repetitions each side
- Wall Control Balance: 8 repetitions each leg
- Wall Open Leg Rocker: 7 repetitions
- Wall Double Leg Stretch: 8 repetitions
- Wall Single Leg Stretch: 8 repetitions each leg
- Wall Spine Stretch Forward: 7 repetitions

Reaching the advanced phase is a testament to your dedication and hard work. Remember to prioritize safety and listen to your body. The advanced exercises are designed to challenge you, but they shouldn't cause pain. Modify as needed, and relish the accomplishments of your Wall Pilates journey!

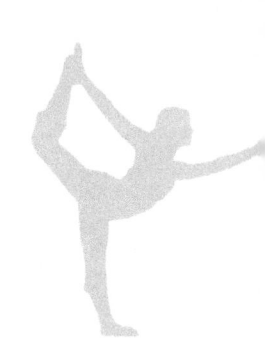

Overcoming Challenges and Embracing Success

Navigating Common Struggles and Frustrations

In every fitness journey, there are inevitable moments of doubt, weariness, and frustration. Wall Pilates, despite its myriad of benefits, is no exception. The very allure of the method – its demand for precision, balance, and control – can sometimes be its most challenging aspect, especially when one's body doesn't immediately "obey" or display the desired results.

Sarah, like many others, often found herself battling with the reflection in the mirror, the silent judge that didn't seem to capture her internal progress. There were days when the wall, rather than being a support, seemed more like an unforgiving barrier, highlighting every misalignment, every tremor of instability.

The initial allure of Wall Pilates can wane when faced with these stark realities. Yet, it's precisely at these crossroads of struggle that true transformation begins. Instead of viewing the wall as an opponent, it's about seeing it as a truthful friend, offering feedback and guidance. The wall doesn't lie; it shows where

your strengths are and where work is still needed.
For Sarah, the turning point came when she began to shift her focus from perfection to progress. Each session became less about the perfect pose and more about listening to her body, understanding its language, and celebrating small victories. She learned to embrace the trembles as signs of muscles awakening and to view each fall or misstep not as a failure but as a lesson.

Moreover, Sarah found solace in knowing she wasn't alone. The Wall Pilates community is filled with stories of women who've faced similar struggles, made mistakes, and found their way back with resilience and determination. By sharing experiences and solutions, they collectively built a network of support and inspiration.

In Wall Pilates, as in life, it's essential to remember that the journey is just as important, if not more so, than the destination. The wall is a constant, always there to support and challenge, reflecting back both our vulnerabilities and our strengths. By navigating these common struggles and frustrations with grace, patience, and perseverance, we not only enhance our physical health but also fortify our mental and emotional resilience. It's about understanding that every challenge faced is a step closer to the person we aspire to be.

Tips and Techniques for Consistency and Motivation

In the midst of a bustling life, filled with commitments and unexpected turns, maintaining a consistent Wall Pilates practice can be a challenge. Sarah knew this all too well. There were mornings when the warmth of her bed seemed far more inviting than the cold embrace of the wall. There were evenings when fatigue whispered tempting excuses, urging her to skip just this once. Yet, over time, she uncovered strategies that kept her tethered to her commitment, ensuring that her motivation burned brightly even on the gloomiest days.

Firstly, Sarah learned the power of intention. Every evening, before drifting off to sleep, she would visualize her morning routine, from the gentle stretching of her muscles to the feeling of accomplishment post-practice. This mental rehearsal not only prepared her body but also aligned her mind, making the transition from thought to action smoother.

Integrating Wall Pilates into her daily life was another game-changer. Rather than seeing it as an 'additional task,' Sarah started incorporating elements of her practice into routine activities. While waiting for her morning coffee to brew, she'd do a quick wall plank. During her favorite TV show's commercial breaks, she'd challenge herself with a Wall Ballet Stretch. By weaving Wall Pilates into the fabric of her day, it became less of a chore and more of a cherished ritual.
Connecting with like-minded individuals played a crucial role too. Sarah joined a virtual Wall Pilates group, where members would share their daily achievements, swap tips, and offer words of encouragement. The camaraderie and shared sense of purpose fueled her drive, reminding her that she was part of a community, a collective journey of transformation.
Finally, Sarah began to document her journey, not just in terms of physical progress but emotional and mental growth too. Reflecting on her thoughts, feelings, and experiences allowed her to recognize patterns, celebrate milestones, and strategize for future challenges. It became a source of inspiration, a tangible reminder of how far she'd come and the potential that lay ahead.

Consistency in Wall Pilates, as Sarah discovered, isn't just about discipline; it's about passion, connection, and a deep-rooted desire to evolve. When we anchor our practice in these values, motivation flows naturally, guiding us through moments of doubt and propelling us towards our goals.

Tracking Your Progress: Journals, Apps, and More

The journey of Wall Pilates is as much about reflection as it is about action. As one delves deeper into this practice, the subtle shifts in strength, flexibility, and posture become evident. But to truly appreciate and navigate this evolution, it's essential to have a system in place that captures the nuances of your progress. Starting with a simple journal can be profoundly impactful. While it might seem traditional in this digital age, the tactile experience of writing can deepen the connection between mind and body. Each evening, take a moment to jot down your Wall Pilates experiences of the day. This might include any new exercises you tried, how they felt, or even the emotions that bubbled up during the practice. Over time, flipping through these pages will reveal a tapestry of growth and change, a chronicle of your journey.

In the digital realm, a plethora of apps are designed specifically for tracking fitness progress. These apps often come equipped with features that allow you to input daily routines, set reminders, and even access guided Wall Pilates sessions. Using visuals, these tools can help pinpoint areas of improvement, offering a dynamic overview of your evolving capabilities.

Moreover, consider the power of visual documentation. Photographs and short video clips can be invaluable. Capture your form during specific exercises, noting the alignment and posture. Over weeks and months, these visual markers will offer a clear representation of your transformation. This visual journey can be incredibly motivating, showcasing not just physical change but the confidence and grace that comes with mastery.

While Wall Pilates is a deeply personal endeavor, don't shy away from sharing your progress with close friends or family. They can provide an external perspective, often noticing changes that you might overlook. Their observations and encouragement can further bolster your commitment.

Ultimately, tracking progress in Wall Pilates is about weaving a narrative of growth. Whether through written reflections, digital tools, or visual documentation, these tracking methods serve as reminders of the journey's beauty, punctuated with moments of challenge, triumph, and profound self-discovery.

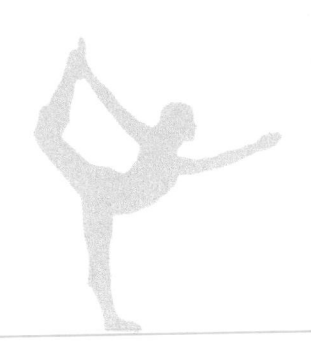

Beyond the Workout – A Holistic Approach

Complementary Diets for Wall Pilates Enthusiasts

Wall Pilates, as a practice, is a harmonious blend of strength, flexibility, and mindfulness. Just as the body and mind intertwine during these exercises, the sustenance we offer our bodies plays a crucial role in optimizing the benefits of this workout. Adopting a complementary diet can enhance performance, speed up recovery, and imbue the practitioner with a sense of holistic well-being.

When embarking on the Wall Pilates journey, the body needs nourishment that supports muscle growth and repair while also fueling the energy required for these exercises. Protein becomes paramount. Incorporating lean sources like chicken, turkey, fish, tofu, and legumes ensures the muscles have the amino acids necessary to repair and grow.

However, it's not just about muscle. Wall Pilates also challenges the connective tissues, requiring a diet rich in collagen or collagen-boosting foods. Bone broths, citrus fruits, berries, and leafy greens are excellent choices, assisting in keeping the joints supple and resilient.

The intricate movements and postures in Wall Pilates demand a sharp, focused mind. Omega-3 fatty acids, found in abundance in fatty fish, chia seeds, and walnuts, can enhance cognitive functions, aiding concentration during sessions.

Hydration is another cornerstone. The body loses fluids during exercise, and replenishing them is vital. But beyond just water, electrolyte-rich foods like bananas, sweet potatoes, and coconut water can help maintain the body's mineral balance, preventing cramps and muscle fatigue.

Lastly, one cannot overlook the role of antioxidants. The physical exertion during Wall Pilates produces free radicals, which, in excess, can hamper recovery. Foods rich in antioxidants, such as berries, dark chocolate, nuts, and green tea, help neutralize these free radicals, ensuring the body remains in a balanced state post-workout.

In embracing Wall Pilates, one is not just adopting a workout but a lifestyle. This lifestyle calls for a diet that resonates with the practice's ethos: balance, strength, and mindfulness. By intertwining the right foods with the exercises, practitioners pave the way for a holistic transformation, where every meal complements the journey on the wall, nourishing both body and soul.

Meditation, Mindfulness, and Wall Pilates

The essence of Wall Pilates isn't merely confined to physical exertion; it's an intertwining of both the mind and body, echoing the centuries-old practices of meditation and mindfulness. When one delves into Wall Pilates, they are not just moving their body but also cultivating a mindset anchored in the present moment.

Meditation, at its core, is the practice of focused attention. Similarly, Wall Pilates demands a deep connection between thought and motion. Each movement, be it a stretch or a hold, requires an acute awareness of the body's positioning, alignment, and sensation. This intimate understanding can only be achieved when one's mind is free from distractions, fully immersed in the act.

Mindfulness, on the other hand, is the art of being wholly present. In our bustling lives, it's all too easy to become lost in thoughts of the past or anxieties of the future. However, Wall Pilates becomes a sanctuary where the external world fades away, and one's entire consciousness is directed towards the nuances of each posture, the rhythm of each breath, and the subtle shifts in energy.

This merger of physical movement with a meditative mindset has profound implications. Stress, often seen as an inevitable byproduct of modern life, begins to dissolve. The focus required in Wall Pilates acts as a natural barrier to intrusive thoughts, giving the mind a much-needed respite. Over time, as one deepens their practice, this tranquil state of mind begins to permeate life outside the workout, imbuing everyday moments with a newfound sense of calm and clarity.

Moreover, the coupling of Wall Pilates with meditation and mindfulness enhances the benefits of the exercise manifold. The mind-body connection is strengthened, resulting in more precise movements, better balance, and an elevated sense of proprioception. This synergy ensures that the practitioner is not just working out but is also engaging in a form of moving meditation.

In essence, Wall Pilates, meditation, and mindfulness are kindred spirits, each amplifying the other's virtues. They together form a trifecta of holistic wellness, nurturing the body, calming the mind, and nourishing the soul. Through this symbiotic relationship, practitioners are offered a path not just to physical prowess but also to inner peace, making Wall Pilates a journey of both external strength and internal serenity.

Connecting with a Community: Workshops, Conferences, and social media

Wall Pilates isn't just an exercise regime; it's a movement, a lifestyle, a passion that connects enthusiasts from all over the world. At its heart, the essence of Wall Pilates thrives on community spirit, allowing practitioners to support, uplift, and inspire each other in their individual journeys.
Workshops play a pivotal role in this. They serve as a hub where novices and veterans alike come together to learn, grow, and share their experiences. Under the guidance of seasoned instructors, these spaces become incubators of knowledge and technique refinement. But more than that, they foster connections, friendships, and bonds that go beyond the confines of the studio. The laughter, the struggles, the shared sense of accomplishment - these are the moments that resonate deeply and form lasting memories.

Conferences, on the other hand, elevate the Wall Pilates experience to a grander scale. Often featuring a lineup of renowned experts, they provide insights into the latest trends, advancements, and best practices in the world of Wall Pilates. But what truly makes these gatherings special is the palpable energy that fills the air. The excitement of meeting like-minded individuals, the exhilaration of witnessing live demonstrations, the pride in being part of a global movement – it's an experience that's both enlightening and heartwarming.

In this digital age, however, one cannot overlook the immense power of social media in building and nurturing communities. Platforms like Instagram, Facebook, and YouTube have become invaluable tools for Wall Pilates enthusiasts. They allow practitioners to showcase their progress, share tips and tricks, seek advice, and even participate in challenges. The beauty of these platforms lies in their accessibility, ensuring that no matter where one is located, they can always be a part of the Wall Pilates family. The stories of triumphs and tribulations, the words of encouragement, the virtual high-fives – they bridge geographical divides and create a tapestry of interconnected souls.

In essence, Wall Pilates is more than just a set of exercises; it's a movement that celebrates unity in diversity. Through workshops, conferences, and social media, practitioners find their tribe, a safe haven where they are celebrated, understood, and loved. In this community, every individual, regardless of their proficiency level, finds a voice, a space to express, and a home to return to, time and again.

Resources & Additional Support

Recommended Reading and Resources

Wall Pilates, like many disciplines, is enriched by a vast expanse of knowledge, both historical and contemporary. For those wishing to delve deeper, there are countless books, articles, and online resources that can provide additional insights. Among the most notable is Joseph Pilates' own written work, detailing the philosophy and techniques that laid the foundation for modern-day Pilates. However, the world of Wall Pilates is ever-evolving, with new perspectives, research, and methodologies emerging regularly. Today's leading instructors and practitioners have contributed immensely, penning guides that range from the intricacies of specific exercises to the broader understanding of the practice's holistic benefits. Moreover, online forums, webinars, and courses are treasure troves of interactive learning, offering both theoretical knowledge and practical demonstrations. Whether you're a beginner or an experienced practitioner, there's always more to explore, learn, and imbibe in this enriching journey of Wall Pilates.

FAQ: Answering the Most Common Wall Pilates Questions

How is Wall Pilates different from traditional Pilates?

While traditional Pilates primarily uses a mat or specialized equipment like the Reformer, Wall Pilates utilizes the wall as a prop. This provides resistance and support, allowing for a unique set of exercises that challenge the body differently and often target posture, alignment, and balance more intensively.

How often should I practice Wall Pilates?

For beginners, starting with two to three times a week is recommended. As you become more accustomed to the exercises and build strength, you can increase the frequency, ensuring you give your body adequate rest between sessions.

What should I do if I experience pain during an exercise?

Listen to your body. If an exercise causes pain, especially sharp or persistent pain, stop immediately.

It's essential to differentiate between the discomfort of a new exercise and actual pain. Always consult with a certified instructor to ensure proper form and seek medical advice if needed.

Is Wall Pilates safe during pregnancy?

While many Pilates exercises can be beneficial during pregnancy, it's essential to consult with a healthcare professional before starting any new exercise regimen. Some Wall Pilates exercises may need modification or should be avoided altogether, depending on the stage of pregnancy and individual health considerations.

Testimonials: Real-life Success Stories

The transformative power of Wall Pilates isn't just encapsulated in theoretical knowledge or technical descriptions; it's most vividly portrayed in the real-life journeys of those who've embraced it. This section is a tribute to those stories.

Meet Elena, a 40-year-old journalist who battled chronic back pain for years. For her, Wall Pilates was more than just a fitness regimen; it was a lifeline. With consistent practice, not only did she alleviate her pain, but she also rediscovered a sense of confidence and joy that had eluded her for so long.

Then there's Jamal, a former athlete who turned to Wall Pilates to rehabilitate after a career-ending injury. Beyond physical recovery, he found mental fortitude and a renewed purpose in life.

These stories, along with countless others, paint a vivid picture of the profound impact Wall Pilates can have. They serve as both inspiration and testimony to the practice's transformative power, echoing the sentiments of countless individuals whose lives have been touched, reshaped, and elevated by Wall Pilates.

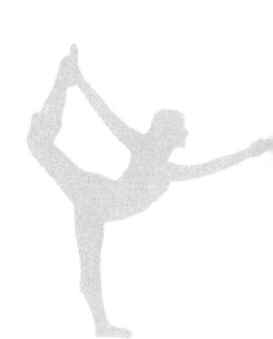

Conclusion

Your Wall Pilates Journey: A Lifetime of Strength, Balance, and Flexibility

The transformative journey you embark upon with Wall Pilates transcends the physical space of your workout area. It's an odyssey that delves deep into the essence of who you are and who you can become. The wall, which you might have once considered just a static part of your home, becomes an active partner in your quest for a healthier, more vibrant self.

As you press your hands, feet, or back against the wall during each exercise, imagine you're pushing against the very challenges and self-imposed limitations that have held you back. Every stretch, every bend, every twist becomes a symbolic and literal release of pent-up tensions, not just from your muscles, but from your psyche.

But Wall Pilates is more than just an exercise regimen. It's a philosophy, a way of viewing your body and your potential in a new light. You'll begin to realize that strength isn't just about muscle size, but about inner resilience. Balance isn't just about not falling over; it's about harmonizing every aspect of your life. Flexibility isn't merely about bending without breaking; it's about adapting and thriving amidst life's constant ebb and flow.

Years down the line, when you reflect on the turning points in your life, your decision to start Wall Pilates will undoubtedly stand out. It's not just about the physical transformations, though they are undoubtedly profound. It's about the mental clarity, the emotional catharsis, and the renewed sense of purpose that comes with aligning body, mind, and soul.

To everyone who embarks on this Wall Pilates journey, know that it's a lifelong commitment to yourself. It's a promise to honor, nurture, and celebrate your body at every stage of life. As you move, stretch, and grow with Wall Pilates, remember that each day brings an opportunity for rebirth, rejuvenation, and rediscovery. Embrace the journey, cherish every moment, and let Wall Pilates guide you toward a lifetime of strength, balance, and flexibility.

Final Words of Encouragement: Every Wall is a New Opportunity

As we close this book and you stand at the threshold of your Wall Pilates journey, remember this pivotal truth: every wall, whether literal or metaphorical, represents a new opportunity. In life, walls often symbolize obstacles, barriers that separate us from our dreams, our goals, and sometimes even from our true selves. Yet, with Wall Pilates, we've turned that narrative on its head. Here, walls are not barriers but bridges, guiding and supporting us as we stretch towards our fullest potential.

It's easy to view challenges as unyielding obstructions. But much like how you've learned to utilize the wall in your workouts, you can transform every challenge you encounter in life. When faced with adversity, don't see a dead-end; envision a wall waiting to be scaled, to be embraced, to be used as a foundation for growth.

The lessons you've absorbed from Wall Pilates go beyond physical postures and exercises. They seep into your psyche, teaching you resilience, persistence, and the art of turning constraints into advantages. Remember, the strength and balance you achieve on the mat (or against the wall) mirror the strength and balance you can achieve in life.

So, as you move forward, let the wall be a constant reminder: In every obstacle, there is an opportunity. In every setback, a lesson. And in every moment of doubt, a chance to push back, to stretch further, to grow stronger.

In Wall Pilates and in life, embrace your walls. Use them, lean on them, grow with them. Because with the right perspective, every wall truly is a new opportunity waiting to be discovered.

I want to thank you for reaching the end and for giving this little manual an opportunity by purchasing it. Do not hesitate to contact me for any reason, or doubt, or advice, or just to say hello. I'll leave you my email address. And if you liked the book and it was useful in any way, leave a vote on Amazon.

Your feedback is valuable and can help me deliver higher quality products.

Thank you for everything!

Liana Sterling

rising2dreamy@gmail.com

Printed in Great Britain
by Amazon